THE

CONSTITUTION AND BY-LAWS

OF THE

MAINE

HOMŒOPATHIC MEDICAL SOCIETY,

LIST OF MEMBERS, Etc.,

1876.

BANGOR:
BURR & ROBINSON, PRINTERS.
1876.

ACT OF INCORPORATION.

STATE OF MAINE.

In the Year of our Lord one thousand eight hundred and sixty-seven.

AN ACT to incorporate the MAINE HOMŒOPATHIC MEDICAL SOCIETY.

Be it enacted by the Senate and House of Representatives in Legislature assembled, as follows:

SECTION 1. W. E. Payne, M. R. Pulsifer, E. Clark, H. B. Eaton, C. H. Burr, W. L. Thompson, N. G. H. Pulsifer, J. M. Blaisdell, J. Esten, M. S. Briry, Geo. R. Clark, B. L. Dresser, N. Wiggin, J. H. Barrows, J. W. Savage, S. H. Boynton, F. A. Roberts, and James B. Bell, and others who may be elected agreeably to the rules and by-laws hereafter to be established, are hereby created a body politic by the name of the Maine Homœopathic Medical Society, with power to sue and be sued, to have a common seal and to change the same, to make any by-laws not repugnant to the laws of this State.

[Approved by the Governor.]

CALL ISSUED

FOR A

MAINE HOMŒOPATHIC MEDICAL SOCIETY.

To...*M. D.*

MY DEAR COLLEAGUE:—I am directed by a vote of the Central Homœopathic Medical Association of Maine, to issue a call to the several members of our School throughout the State, to meet in Convention at the City Council Room, Augusta, the 3d TUESDAY of January, proximo, at 10 o'clock, A. M., for the purpose of organizing a State Society.

The interests of Homœopathy in this State seem to demand an organization of this kind, and the general sentiment of the profession favors the present time. It is to be hoped, therefore, that nothing but necessity will keep you away from the proposed meeting.

It is proposed to hold an adjourned meeting of the CENTRAL HOMŒOPATHIC MEDICAL ASSOCIATION OF MAINE, at the same place, immediately after the State organization is effected, in the deliberations of which you are hereby invited to take an active part.

Please favor me with an early reply.

Fraternally yours, WM. E. PAYNE,
Pres. Me. Cen. Hom. Assoc.

BATH, Dec. 24th, 1866.

Pursuant to the foregoing call there was holden at Augusta, in the City Council Room, on the 15th day of January, 1867, a meeting composed of the following members of the Homœopathic profession of Maine, viz.:

WM. E. PAYNE, Bath,	M. R. PULSIFER, Ellsworth,
CHAS. H. BURR, Portland,	M. S. BRIRY, Bath,
JAS. W. SAVAGE, Wiscasset,	NATHAN WIGGIN, Rockland,
JOHN ESTEN, Rockland,	GEO. R. CLARK, Portland,
JAS. B. BELL, Augusta,	WM. L. THOMPSON, Augusta,
S. H. BOYNTON, Skowhegan,	H. B. EATON, Rockport,
F.A.ROBERTS,No.Vassalboro,'	J. H. BARROWS, Gardiner,
B. L. DRESSER, Searsport,	J. M. BLAISDELL, Bangor,

N. G. H. PULSIFER, Waterville.

The convention was called to order by Dr. N. G. H. Pulsifer, of Waterville, and Dr. M. R. Pulsifer, of Ellsworth, was chosen by the convention temporary chairman, and Dr. James B. Bell, temporary secretary.

Prayer was offered by the Rev. D. B. Randall, of Augusta, for which the convention passed him a vote of thanks.

Drs. Thompson, Burr, Eaton, Esten and Blaisdell, were appointed a committee by the chair to nominate permanent officers.

Drs. Payne, Bell, Burr, Dresser and Boynton, were appointed a committee to report a constitution and by-laws to the convention.

The committee made a report of the following constitution and by-laws, which were adopted by the convention.

CONSTITUTION

OF THE

MAINE HOMŒOPATHIC MEDICAL SOCIETY.

ARTICLE I.—Name.

This Association shall be known by the name of the MAINE HOMŒOPATHIC MEDICAL SOCIETY.

ARTICLE II.—Object.

The object of this Society shall be the cultivation of the science and art of medicine, the promotion of friendly intercourse between its members, and of greater harmony of action among them.

ARTICLE III.—Members.

This Society shall consist of those physicians who may become members of this organization, and also all those Homœopathic physicians of the State of Maine, who may be hereafter duly elected in conformity with its by-laws.

ARTICLE IV.—Officers.

The officers of this Society shall consist of a president, two vice-presidents, a corresponding secretary, a recording secretary and a treasurer, with such other officers as may be designated by the by-laws; to be chosen at such a time, and in such a manner, and for such a period, and with such duties as those by-laws shall ordain.

ARTICLE V.—Seal.

This Society shall have and use one common seal, with such a device and inscription as the Society in its deliberative capacity shall determine.

ARTICLE VI.—Alteration or Amendment.

This constitution may be altered or amended by a vote of two-thirds of all the members present at any regular annual meeting, provided that notice of such alteration or amendment shall have been given in writing, at a previous annual meeting of this Society.

BY-LAWS.

I. The Maine Homœopathic Medical Society shall hold one session annually, at such time and place as may be determined upon by the Society from time to time, and a special meeting of the Society shall be called by the president whenever eight members shall make a written request, setting forth, therein the object of said meeting, which object shall be stated in the notice sent out to the members, and no other business shall be transacted at such special meeting than that embraced in the call and notice, as issued to the several members.

II. The officers of this Society shall be a president, two vice-presidents, a corresponding secretary, a recording secretary, a treasurer, and five censors, who, together, shall constitute an executive committee, to whom shall be intrusted the general business of the Society, when not in session, and shall be elected annually by ballot, and a majority of all the votes shall be necessary to a choice, and each of the officers above named shall continue in office till the adjournment of the annual meeting next after their election, at which time the duties of the newly elected officers shall commence. The general duties of the officers shall be as herein prescribed.

III. The president shall preside at all meetings of the Society and of the executive committee, taking the chair at the appointed hour—call the members to order, cause the roll of membership to be called, and so much of the journal of preceding meeting to be read as relates to unfinished business. He shall preserve order and conduct the business of the meeting according to accepted parliamentary rules. He shall deliver an address before the Society at the commencement of the next annual meeting after his election. He shall appoint all committees not otherwise ordered, and direct the recording secretary to call extra meetings when required, as provided by the first section of the by-laws.

IV. The vice-presidents shall preside in the absence of the president, and in case the office of president shall become vacant, they shall perform the duties of that office until the next succeeding election, the senior officer taking the precedence. In the absence of both president and vice-presidents, the senior censor shall preside, or should all those officers be absent, the Society may choose a chairman to preside at said meeting.

V. The corresponding secretary shall have charge and custody of all letters and communications addressed to the Society, conduct the necessary correspondence, and in the absence of the recording secretary, he shall discharge the duties devolving upon that officer.

VI. It shall be the duty of the recording secretary to give proper and timely notice of the meetings; keep a record of all the proceedings of the Society; notify members of their election; sign, in conjunction with the president, certificates of membership and diplomas; record the names of members, date of admission and other required particulars; preserve all papers delivered to him, and allow none at any time to pass out of his hands, except by the direction of the Society; he shall notify the chairman of all committees appointed by the Society, of his appointment, stating the commission and the names of the committee, and at the close of his term of office, he shall deliver the records and other papers belonging to the Society into the hands of his successor in office.

VII. It shall be the duty of the treasurer to receive and keep all moneys belonging to the Society and pay all bills after they shall have been approved by the executive committee. He shall keep an accurate account of all receipts and expenditures and submit his account with vouchers for all expenditures at each annual meeting, which account shall be audited by a committee on the treasurer's accounts, chosen by the Society.

VIII. It shall be the duty of the censors to receive and examine the credentials of all applicants for membership, and report to the Society for election, all such persons for election as may be found properly qualified according to the requirements of the by-laws. (Addenda, May, 1876.) And the censors shall report to the Society the Medical College and date of graduation of each successful applicant from which he received his diploma, which shall be recorded by the secretary if admitted to membership. The censors shall be in session at each annual meeting, three of whom shall constitue a quorum.

IX. Any person shall be eligible to membership who has received the degree of Doctor of Medicine from a legally authorized medical institution, sustains a good moral character, and acknowledges and practices medicine according to the law *Similia Similibus Curantur*, and having been examined and approved by the board of censors, he shall be elected by ballot at the annual meeting, and become a member of the

Society by signing the by-laws.

(Addenda, May, 1868,) And paying into the treasury the sum of two dollars as an admission fee; and one dollar as an annual tax at each annual session for the current year in advance.

X. It shall be the duty of each member of the Society to make a written or verbal communication at every annual meeting, having a practical bearing on the interest of Homœopathy, and make every reasonable effort to attend punctually all the meetings of the Society, and assist in making them useful and interesting.

XI. Any member of this Society shall forfeit his membership and be expelled therefrom by a vote of two-thirds of the members present at any regular meeting, on the substantiation of either of the following charges, provided he shall have had due notice, through, or by direction of the executive committee, of the charges preferred, and the time and place where such charges are to be investigated, and thereby had opportunity afforded him to appear before the Society and speak in his own defence:

First. For any gross immorality, habitual intemperance, or the perpetration of any crime against the laws of the country, and the abetting thereof.

Second. For any attempt to subvert the object or injure the reputation and standing of this Society, or any member thereof.

Third. For an attempt to enhance his individual interests, and injure scientific medicine by advertising, vending or pretending to a knowledge and use of any secret nostrums.

Fourth. For making a false representation either in his own behalf or that of any student of medicine, or any aspirant to membership of this Society, thereby attempting to secure undeservedly positions of eminence by professional endorsements.

Fifth. For habitually holding professional consultations with persons who practice medicine without the professional acquirements necessary to entitle them to the confidence of the members of this Society.

Sixth. (Addenda, May, 1872.) By refusing or neglecting to pay the annual tax or assessment of one dollar for each year, unless excused by vote of the Society.

XII. There shall be chosen by ballot at each annual meeting two delegates to represent this Society in the next succeeding meeting of the American Institute of Homœopathy, and such delegates shall be furnished with certificates of their election by the recording secretary.

XIII. All papers read before, and communications addressed to this Society shall become its property, but no paper shall be published as a part of the transactions except by a vote of the Society; nor shall the reception or publication by this Society of any paper be considered as an endorsement of its sentiments.

XIV. The presiding officer shall preserve order in the meetings of the Society according to parliamentary rules. The following shall be the order of business:

First. Calling the roll of members.

Second. Annual address by the president.

Third. Reading so much of the minutes of the last meeting as relates to unfinished business, or matters refered to the next meeting.

Fourth. Appointment of committees on treasurer's account.

Fifth. Report of treasurer, with vouchers of expenditures.

Sixth. Report of committees appointed at the last meeting.

Seventh. Balloting for new members.

Eighth. Reading of papers and miscellaneous business.

Ninth. Informal convention on scientific subjects.

Tenth. Choice of officers for the ensuing year.

Eleventh. Choice of delegates to American Institute of Homœopathy.

Twelfth. Reading the minutes for correction and approval.

Thirteenth. Time and place of next meeting, and committee of arrangements.

Fourteenth. Adjournment.

The above order may be varied or suspended for the time, by common consent, or by a vote of two-thirds of the members present.

XV. The established fee bills of physicians in the vicinity of members of this Society shall govern their charges for services, but may be reduced from inability to pay the regular fee. But it shall be considered dishonorable to diminish the standard fees with a view to mercenary competition; but gratuitous services to the poor are always commendable.

XVI. These by-laws may be altered or amended by a vote of a majority of the members present, at any annual meeting of the Society.

LIST OF MEMBERS.

Wm. E. Payne, M. M.,	Bath.
James B. Bell, M. D.,	Augusta.
Eliphalet Clark, M. D.,	Portland.
Charles H. Burr, M. D.,	Portland.
Sumner H. Boynton, M. D.,	Rockland.
†John Estin, M. D.	Rockland.
Hosea B. Eaton, M. D.,	Rockport.
Moses Dodge, M. D.,	Portland.
Milton S. Briry, M. D.,	Bath.
* George R. Clark, M. D.,	Portland.
Charles A. Cochran, M. D.,	Winthrop.
H. C. Bradford, M. D.,	Lewiston.
Thomas L. Bradford, M. D.,	Skowhegan.
* J. W. Barrows, M. D.,	Hallowell.
John M. Blaisdell, M. D.,	Bangor.
† Dr. Benj. L. Dresser,	Searsport.
David P. Flanders, M. D.,	Belfast.
† Ivory S. Hall, M. D.,	Hallowell.
† G. H. Morrill, M. D.,	Augusta.
† Frederick W. Payne, M. D.,	Bath.
Moses R. Pulsifer, M. D.,	Ellsworth.
N. G. H. Pulsifer, M. D.,	Waterville.
Francis A. Roberts, M. D.,	No. Vassalboro.
Rufus Shackford, M. D.,	Portland.
Wm. L. Thompson, M. D.,	Augusta.
Geo. P. Thompson, M. D.,	Portland.
* Rufus R. Williams, M. D.,	Gardiner.
Dr. Nathan Wiggin,	Rockland.
William Gallupe, M. D.,	Bangor.

George P. Jefferds, M. D.,	Bangor.
S. P. Graves, M. D.,	Saco.
† Dr. Edward S. Hincks,	Thomaston.
J. W. Savage, M. D.,	Wiscasset.
George A. Clark, M. D.,	Portland.
† James B. Robinson, M. D.,	Gardiner.
D. E. Seymour, M. D.,	Calais.
Wm. Waters, M. D.,	Mechanic Falls.
Olin M. Drake, M. D.,	Ellsworth.
† Thomas B. Pulsifer, M. D.,	Bangor.
* John L. Babcock, M. D.,	Gardiner.
David S. Richards, M. D.,	Richmond.
James S. Gannett, M. D.,	Waterville.
Daniel C. Perkins, M. D.,	No. Vassalboro.
* Henry Waters, M. D.,	Mechanic Falls.
David N. Skinner, M. D.,	Auburn.
Wm. K. Knowles, M. D.,	Searsport.
Rodolph Lorenzo Dodge,	Portland.
Wesley B. Perkins, M. D.,	Portland.
Silas C. Sylvester, M. D.,	Portland.
Wm. Frank Shepard, M. D.,	Bangor.

* Died. † Removed from the State.

www.ingramcontent.com/pod-product-compliance
Lightning Source LLC
LaVergne TN
LVHW010833120826
845149LV00016B/1359
9781418190583